Placental Histopathological Manifestations and their Relevance to Foetal and Maternal Outcomes

Asokaplus

Placental Histopathological Manifestations and their Relevance to Foetal and Maternal Outcomes

Dr. S.B. Asoka Dissanayake; M.B.B.S (Ceylon)

Asokaplus

Asokaplus

Disclaimer

Author does not claim that this study as comprehensive but only complementary to examination of the newborn

Asokaplus

Table of Contents

Abstract..11

Study Design to Critically Examine Microscopic Morphological Features of the Placenta in Relation to Clinical Entities (Maternal Nutrition, Pregnancy Induced Hypertension and Prematurity) with Special Reference to Intrauterine Growth Restriction of Sri-Lankan Newborns 11

1. Introduction...13
   - *Sri-Lankan Perspective and Why Present Study?*..14
2. Objectives 16
3. Hypothesis...17
4. Sample:..17
5. Methods...17
   - *Morphometry*...18
   - *Accuracy and Precision of Morphometry*..18
   - *Recording Macroscopic Features*..19
   - *Defining the 10th centile for Maternal BMI*..20
   - *Defining Growth Restricted Infants (IUGR)*...20
   - *Defining I.U.G.R Categories*...20
   - *Defining Poor Maternal Nutrition*..20
   - *a) Defining Normal Placentae for Histological Examination*...........................21
   - *b) Defining Abnormal Placentae for Histological Examination*.......................21
   - *Defining Abnormal Macroscopic Morphological Categories*..........................21

A. Quantitative Assessment..22
   - *Defining Microscopic Categories / Entities Observed Under Light Microscope* 22
     - a. Groping of Blood Vessels for the assessment of their Dimensions................22
     - b. Defining Terminal Chorionic Villous Tissue 22
   - *The Amount of Stromal Tissue*...23
   - *Syncytial Knots* 23
   - *Deposition of Fibrin like Material-Fibrinoid Change*.......................................23
   - *Avascular TCV*..24
   - *Other microscopic Features (infarction, fibrosis and calcification)*..................24

B. Qualitative Assessment 24

C. Clinical and Pathological Categories analyze..24

D. Gestational Age as an independent variable..25

E. Study of morphological features in relation to clinical entities. Objective analysis of placental microscopic features in relation to maternal illnesses, poor maternal

nutrition and foetal outcomes were attempted, having collected placental, foetal and maternal data from a random sample of mothers. 25
6. Results...26
    Statistics on Maternal BMI and Foetal BMI...26
        1. Mean BMI in the Second Half of Pregnancy.................................26
        2. Determination of BMI value, 2 Standard Deviations below the Mean value for Gestational Age (for Premature and Term Newborn Infants)...............26
    Determinants of Growth Retardation / Restriction (I.U.G.R) according Maturity. 26
        3. Percentage of different I.U.G.R Categories (of the total, according to Intra Uterine Growth Restriction defined) 26
        4. Disparities observed between the Clinical Parameters and the actual number of Growth Restricted Newborns detected..27
        5. Low Birth Weight with Intrauterine Growth Retardation / Restriction..........27
        6. Premature Infants...28
        7. Relationship of Measured Morphological Entities of the Placenta with Gestation..28
8. Inter Category Relationships of Histological and Histopathological Entities................29
    1. Amount of Villus Stroma..29
    2. Syncytial knots 30
    3. Deposition of Fibrin- Fibrinoid Change...30
    4. Avascular T.C.V...31
    5. Fibrosis...31
    6. Calcification..31
    7. Infarction..32
Relationship of Microscopic Features with Clinical Condition..32
    1. Prematurity...32
    2. Dysmature Placenta...33
    3. Low Maternal BMI..34
    4. P.I.H...36
7. Discussion...37
    1. Defining Growth Restricted Infants..37
    2. Defining Poor Maternal Nutrition...37
    3. Defining Categories of I.U.G.R..38
    4. Low Birth Weight Infants..39
Placental Morphological Findings..40
    Villous Dimensions 40
    Microscopic Entities and their associations and relationships..........................41
        1. Amount of Villus Stroma...41
        2. Syncytial Knots..41
        3. Deposition of Fibrin like Material- Fibrinoid Change................................42
        4. Avascular Terminal Villi..46

        5. Fibrosis..49
        6. Infarction..49
        7. Calcification...50
Qualitative Features...51
    Associations of Microscopic Features with Clinical entities..............52
        1. Findings in PIH...52
        2. Findings in Low Maternal BMI..52
        3. Findings in Dysmature Placenta..52
        4. Findings in Premature Infants...53
8. Conclusions...54
    A. *Validity of Foetal and Maternal BMI*....................................54
    B. *Validity of Histopathological Entities*..................................54
    Future Studies..59
    Chart 1..61
    Chart 2..63
    Chart 3..65
    Chart 4..67
    Chart 5..69
    Chart 6..71
    Chart 7..73
    Chart 8..75
    Chart 9..77
    Chart 10..79
    Chart 11..81
    Chart 12..83
    Image 1...85
    Image 2...87
    Image 3...89
    Image 4...91
    Image 5...93
    Image 6...95
    Image 7...97
    Image 8...99
    Image 9...101
    Image10..103
    References...105
    Appendix I..111
    Appendix II...115
    Authors Note...123

Abstract

Study Design to Critically Examine Microscopic Morphological Features of the Placenta in Relation to Clinical Entities (Maternal Nutrition, Pregnancy Induced Hypertension and Prematurity) with Special Reference to Intrauterine Growth Restriction of Sri-Lankan Newborns

Dr. S.B.Asoka Dissanayake M.B.B.S (Ceylon)

Asokaplus

1. Introduction

Placenta is essentially a vascular tissue but with a difference.

It has unique evolutionary behaviour with two distinct circulations one maternal and the other foetal interposed between a syncytium of trophoblastic (haemochorial) tissue which act as the inter-phase between the mother and the foetus [11] (***Beconsfield P, Birdwood G, Beconsfield R; 1996***). The complex relationship of these circulations cannot be studied one independent of the other. When placenta separates from the basal plate at delivery only a few fragments of maternal blood vessels are left intact with the placenta. Maternal blood vessels can be studied by placental bed biopsy but the present study does not entail such an endeavour.

Broadly speaking placental development is determined by genetic, environmental, vascular and unknown factors. Genetic factors cannot be manipulated but environmental (nutrition) and vascular (pharmacological) factors are theoretically amenable to manipulation. Studies [47,49] (***Winick M and Noble A; 1966***) have shown that in rats with intrauterine growth retardation without gross malformations there was proportionate reduction of placental weight and of protein content but had increase in RNA content. Protein / DNA ratios were normal for the size of the placenta but the RNA/DNA ratios were markedly elevated. These data indicated that in intrauterine growth retardation there was an association of reduced placental weight accompanied by reduced number of cells. The increase in RNA content was a manifest response to the placental insufficiency. For the first time their studies had shown that the small placentae of intrauterine growth retarded rats were functionally different. Whether this response is pathological or physiological was not clear from their studies but the difference of functional activity was shown. Enhanced expression of RNA may be an indication of metabolic response to stress. Whether these RNA products result in advanced placental maturation with short term survival advantage (epigenetic phenomenon) to the infant or premature expression of biological components that modify the arterial structure that leads to hypertension in adult life are contemporary issues.

[21]**Emanuel et al** have shown increased ACTH levels in maternal blood and amniotic fluids in mothers with PIH. These findings were coincident with increased syncytial knots. Syncytial knots are not normally seen until 35 weeks of gestation and are generally considered to relate to the maturity of the placenta. In patients with PIH and placental insufficiency, an associated increased production of ACTH, an increase in number of syncytial knots and advanced placental maturation were noted by these researchers. Increased cortisol production [30,31](**Lindsay RS, Lindsay RM, Edwards CRW; 1996**) in placenta in intrauterine life has been associated with development of hypertension in juvenile rats.

Sri-Lankan Perspective and Why Present Study?

The relationship of the microscopic placental features that are frequently observed when examined by a pathologist is not determined for even a normally grown infant at birth in Sir-Lanakn context. It is difficult to say whether a particular finding detected when examined is normal or abnormal, let alone their clinical significance. The potential of the placental pathological features in the assessment of growth compromised infants, too is ill defined. Histological features that identify intrauterine insults that retard fetal growth need defining for our infants. Furthermore, the relevance of histopathological features to prematurity, Low Birth Weight infant (as defined by WHO criterion of 2.5 Kg and under) and adverse pregnancy outcomes need evaluating.

Even though, the effect is retrospective, the examination of the placenta morphologically at the time of the birth is a scientific exercise. One cannot study all the aspects of clinical significance in a single study. but this is an attempt to untangle, the tangled mysteries of the placenta in a sample of Sri-Lankan infants born in a tertiary setup.

While there is major clinical interest in the West to the potential benefits of placental examination, in Sri-Lankan context there is paucity of standardized histological data relevant to placenta of our infants.

Furthermore, maturity of infant is ill defined and WHO classification of underweight (below 2500 gm) is universally accepted as a standard for growth restriction without critical analysis.

With this in mind standardization of placental histological data with special reference to gestational age was undertaken. Once standardized, an objective analysis was undertaken. For these histological data to be meaningful in clinical and scientific use objective reference to maternal and foetal outcome was necessary.

How these data compare with international findings need evaluating with special reference to Intrauterine Growth Restriction of our infants.

2. Objectives

Both *quantitative* and *qualitative* analysis were considered necessary prerequisites for detailed placental examination at the time of delivery. In addition how each element of examination relate to defined categories would be observed, wherever it was objectively feasible.

a) Evaluation of Placental Histological Features and estimation of the changing histological patterns with advancing gestation age was the *Primary Objective*.

b) Identifying histopathological features that indicate Intrauterine Growth Restriction (IUGR) and defining histopathological injuries associated with Pregnancy Induced Hypertension (PIH), Poor Maternal Nutrition (PMN) and various pregnancy related clinical entities were the *Secondary Objectives*.

c) Histological features observed were classified according to their appearance under the microscope, the size and distribution of these histological entities were examined. In addition, the foetal vasculature and their size and presence or absence of foetal vessels in placental villi were studied.

3. Hypothesis

Placental examination at the time of delivery of the newborn infant is relevant to maternal and foetal wellbeing. Furthermore, microscopic placental features can be detected at the time of delivery and they can be defined histopathologically and they in turn identify clinical entities and intrauterine growth restriction of newborns.

4. Sample:

A random sample of 316 mothers, newborn infants and their placentae were examined

5. Methods

New developments in histological methods of investigations and in therapy (e. g, non-Hodgkin's lymphoma) have increased the need for more accurate identification and improved reproducibility in diagnostic histopathology. In tissue pathology, reproducibility [17](***Collan Y***; Reproducibility, neglected cornerstone of medical diagnosis). In ***Collan Y, Romppanen T,*** eds. Morphometry in Morphological diagnosis. Kuopio: Kuopio University Press, 1982) must be considered before accuracy or specificity. Accurate classification or diagnosis can only be achieved if reproducible methods are used to evaluate histological criteria. Poor reproducibility means there is either subjective bias or the methodology is defective.

Morphometry

Morphometry (the measurements of form) is an objective and reproducible procedure which can be used to measure and interpret tissue features and assist the diagnosis when subjective evaluation is difficult and gives indefinite results. Morphometry of 2 dimensional tissue sections can also be used to provide information on the 3 dimensional spatial structure or organization (referred to as stereology) of tissue. Stereology and morphometry are closely related and often used interchangeably.

Visual perceptions do not always reproduce physical reality.

This is due to the illusory effects when viewing histological sections, as the tissue architecture or structures in which cells are located or surrounded can lead to errors in perceptual judgment. This is especially true in placenta due to complex arborization of **Terminal Chorionic Villi** and their arrangement in relation to the inter-villous space.

Accuracy and Precision of Morphometry

Precision describes the repeatability of a measurement. Accuracy, on the other hand is the assessed as the difference between the measured and known value. Accuracy can only be assessed if independent certification of the true answer is possible, such as by measuring known standards or identifying all bias in the measurement. To improve the accuracy of the estimate it would be necessary to collect more data. That is to increase the number of samples and the sample size.

Sampling error is of considerable importance in designing a morphometric study. To minimize the sampling errors statistical methods have to be used in designing.

Recording Macroscopic Features

Placental examination was undertaken in accordance of the "Practice Guideline for Examination of the placenta by [29]**Langston C, Kaplan T, Macpherson et al, of 1997.** Unusual macroscopic features were noted and their sites were recorded in a line diagram. Placenta was palpated for its softness, firmness and grittiness and the palpable features were recorded as soft or firm or fibrous or gritty (sandy).

The placenta was sectioned in a "bread loaf fashion" (perpendicular to the foetal surface) at approximately 1 to 2 cm intervals and cut slices were examined for any abnormality. Representative samples were taken from what appeared normal at least $1/3^{rd}$ distance form the periphery of the placenta. An additional piece of placenta horizontal to the decidual surface (maternal surface) was sampled. Samples of macroscopically abnormal placental tissues were taken, marked with "x" for identification. Fixed samples (formalin) of cord, membrane rolls and chorionic tissues were trimmed (divided to fit the cassettes) and were embedded for histological examination. Microscopic assessment we based broadly on [26,27]***Kilman et all*** descriptions (syncytil knots and fibrinoid change) but additional parameters were included (amount of stromal tissue in villi, definition of Terminal Villi on the basis of number of blood vessels) exclusively in this study.

Defining the 10th centile for Maternal BMI

Maternal BMI in the second half of the pregnancy was estimated from maternal weight, height data and the 10th centile was determined as the cut off point of poor maternal nutrition.

Defining Growth Restricted Infants (IUGR)

Foetal BMI, two standard deviations below the mean according to gestational age was utilized to define the intrauterine growth restricted newborns.

Defining I.U.G.R Categories

Five categories of Intra Uterine Growth Restriction were determined and they included I.U.G.R due to P.I.H, I.U.G.R associated with clinically silent macroscopic placental abnormalities *(defined as placental Dysmaturity)*, poor maternal nutrition category *(defined as BMI <20 in the Second Half of Pregnancy)*, due to assortment of antenatal conditions (multiple pregnancy, maternal heart disease, congenital abnormalities) and the cause unknown category

Defining Poor Maternal Nutrition

Both prospective (low maternal BMI) and retrospective (inappropriately low foetal BMI having excluded other causes of I.U.G.R) parameters were utilized to define poor maternal nutrition.

a) Defining Normal Placentae for Histological Examination

All placentae with morphological or abnormal clinical or perinatal conditions were excluded before histological examination. The remaining placentae were defined as normal.

b) Defining Abnormal Placentae for Histological Examination

All placentae with morphological or abnormal clinical or perinatal conditions were defined as abnormal.

Defining Abnormal Macroscopic Morphological Categories

The macroscopic morphological features defined were abnormal insertion of cord or membranes, abnormal shape, macroscopic abnormalities both gross and minor (infarction, fibrosis, antepartum and peripartum haemorrhage), inappropriately small or large placenta.

A. Quantitative Assessment

Defining Microscopic Categories / Entities Observed Under Light Microscope

a. Groping of Blood Vessels for the assessment of their Dimensions.

Blood vessels were grouped into three categories, those <15µ (terminal villi), those between 25 to 75µ (tertiary villous stems) and those > 100µ (secondary villous stems).

b. Defining Terminal Chorionic Villous Tissue

Because of the unresolved controversies regarding the basic placental unit and complex arborizing subdivisions of the villous stems, a need for simple classification of the terminal villi was felt. Micrometer measurement of the terminal villous and a count of its component blood vessels were made. Average diameter of the terminal villous in two perpendicular planes was measured along with the count of the number of blood vessels. The villi were grouped according to number of blood vessels from 1 to 10. Diameters of the blood vessels were measured to avoid examining cut sections of the stem villi which have larger diameter blood vessels. Villi between 40 to 70 microns in size and consisting 4 to 6 foetal blood vessels were defined as terminal.

The Amount of Stromal Tissue

Quantifying the amount of stromal tissue supporting villous blood vessels in cut sections was difficult. To address this, the amount of stromal tissue was grouped according to diameters of the TCV with four foetal blood vessels. Groups were classified from 1 to 7 according to the diameter of the *Terminal Chorionic Villi*.

Syncytial Knots

Syncytial knots are aggregations of multiple syncytial trophoblast (nuclear material) nuclei that form buds at the periphery of the villous surface and can be identified easily under high power magnification. Number of syncytial knots per high power field (at 10 x 40) of magnification was counted in four separate fields and the average count was determined.

Deposition of Fibrin like Material-Fibrinoid Change

Fibrin like material is universally present in the basal plate, in the chorionic plate and in chorionic villi. This material is an acellular mass of dense eosinophilic material that often appears as a lump on the trophoblast basement membrane and is covered completely or partially by syncytiotrophoblastic epithelium. How they form is not very well understood. General belief is that fibrinoid material is formed from both maternal and foetal components. Whether its formation is physiological or pathological is also not known. Deposition of fibrin like material in terminal villi was grouped. Groups were no deposition, minimal (1), mild (2), moderate (3), focal extensive (4), diffuse (5) and diffuse extensive (6) under low power field (at 10 x 10) of magnification. Diameters of the villi with complete fibrin deposition were measured. Fibrin calcification was recorded as present or absent.

Avascular TCV

Avascular Terminal Chorionic Villi (villi with stromal tissue but without blood vessels) were examined and recorded for their presence or absence and their diameters were measured. They were classified into 7 groups according to their diameter. They were also classified into 2 groups according to whether they were associated with other histopathological features or not.

Other microscopic Features (infarction, fibrosis and calcification)

Additional microscopic morphological features grouped and assessed were infarction, fibrosis and calcification.

B. Qualitative Assessment

Qualitative changes were described as congestion, oedema, endarteritis, smooth muscle hypertrophy of larger blood vessels and thrombosis.

C. Clinical and Pathological Categories analyze

Clinical conditions analyzed were P.I.H and the category of low maternal B.M.I (as defined as B.M.I <20). An additional pathological category named as placental Dysmaturity (growth retardation with clinically silent macroscopic placental abnormalities) was defined. Prematurity was analyzed as a clinical category.

D. Gestational Age as an independent variable

Gestational age as an independent variable of placental pattern of histological maturation was studied.

E. Study of morphological features in relation to clinical entities. Objective analysis of placental microscopic features in relation to maternal illnesses, poor maternal nutrition and foetal outcomes were attempted, having collected placental, foetal and maternal data from a random sample of mothers.

Abnormal morphological features both macroscopic and microscopic were defined with the intention of analyzing them against the background of normal growth and growth restriction of the newborn.

6. Results

Statistics on Maternal BMI and Foetal BMI

1. Mean BMI in the Second Half of Pregnancy.

> The mean BMI in the second half of pregnancy was 23.76 ± 3.48.
> The 10th centile was 20.09.

2. Determination of BMI value, 2 Standard Deviations below the Mean value for Gestational Age (for Premature and Term Newborn Infants)

Determinants of Growth Retardation / Restriction (I.U.G.R) according Maturity.

> Foetal BMI less than 10.5 was the cut off point that defined intra-uterine growth retardation of infants between 37 to 42 weeks of gestation. For infants between 36 to 37 weeks of gestation foetal BMI below 10 identified all growth retarded infants. 11% of the mothers were identified as having growth restricted infants (34).

3. Percentage of different I.U.G.R Categories (of the total, according to Intra Uterine Growth Restriction defined)

> Only 17.5% of the infants (2% of the total) could be defined as purely nutritionally deficient out of 34 growth retarded infants (defined according to gestation) due to various etiologies. Placental factors (3.2% of the total) determining growth retardation was 29%. 21% was due to P.I.H (2.3% of the total). 17.5% was

due to various (2% of the total) maternal and foetal conditions (congenital abnormalities, maternal heart disease and multiple pregnancies). 15% was undetermined (1.5 % of the total).

In altogether, 44% of the total (5% of the total) the growth retardation of the newborn was undetermined.

4. Disparities observed between the Clinical Parameters and the actual number of Growth Restricted Newborns detected.

Only 6 (26%) out of 23 infants in whose mothers the maternal B.M.I was below 20 at delivery had significant growth restriction. The combination of placental pathologies increased the number (70%) of affected infants to 16. Only 9 (25%) out of 36 infants whose mother had P.I.H had significant growth restriction. 7 mothers of premature newborns had associated P.I.H. The combination of placental morphological features (those associated with P.I.H) increased the number (20) of affected infants to 55%.

However, 76% of the growth restricted infants had macroscopically detectable placental pathology.

5. Low Birth Weight with Intrauterine Growth Retardation / Restriction

When WHO cut off point of 2500 gm was utilized to group infants into Low Birth Weight category without any qualification to gestational age there were 57 infants with low birth weights. 30 out of 34 infants categorized as growth retarded were included in Low Birth Weight infants. Four (4) infants who were growth restricted but were above 2500 gm were not included.

14 premature (70%) and 13 term (30%) infants with appropriate foetal B.M.I were included in the Low Birth Weight infants. 75% of the Low Birth Weight (L.B.W) infants had macroscopically detectable placental pathology. Altogether 56% did not have any associated clinical condition.

6. Premature Infants

There were 19 premature infants and 6 of them had associated antenatal conditions (mainly P.I.H). Premature infants with appropriate weight (15) for length and gestation were roughly 5% of the total sample. Premature infants with inappropriate weight (4 infants) for length (foetal B.M.I) were roughly 1%.

In only one premature infant the birth weight was above 2500 gm.

7. Relationship of Measured Morphological Entities of the Placenta with Gestation.

The gestational age ($r=0.328$ and $p< 0.006$) had significant relationship with amount of stromal tissues in terminal villi with four blood vessels up to 40 weeks of gestation. Abundance of avascular terminal villi had significant positive relationship with gestation ($r= 0.251$ and $p<0.018$) when all pathological conditions where included in the analysis and also when all the pathological condition were excluded from the sample ($r= 0.414$ and $p<0.029$) was examined.

The number of syncytial knots per high power field did not correlate with gestational age (r=0.226 and p>0.062) up to 40 weeks of gestation in placentae defined as normal.

8. Inter Category Relationships of Histological and Histopathological Entities

1. Amount of Villus Stroma

There was negative correlation of amount of stromal tissues to syncytial knots (r=-0.461 and p<0.001), terminal villous fibrinoid change (r=-0.205 and p<0.028), calcification of fibrin (r=-0.147 and p<0.02) and fibrosis (r=-0.299 and p<0.002). There was no significant correlation of amount of stromal tissues to calcification of stroma (r=-0.149 and p>0.117) and infarction (r=-0.034 and p>0.616). Qualitative changes like villous oedema (r=0.185 and p <0.013) had positive correlation whereas endarteritis (r=-0.248 and p<0.001) displayed negative correlation with the amount of stromal tissue content of the villous.

Gestational age did not have any relationship (total sample) but as shown above when all pathological conditions where excluded (as defined as normal placenta) gestational age had significant relationship (r=0.328 and p < 0.006) up to 40 weeks of gestation.

Blood pressure did not have any relationship with the abundance of stromal tissue.

2. Syncytial knots

Number of syncytial knots correlated negatively with amount of stroma (r=-0.461 and p<0.001), villous dimensions (r=-0.501 and p<0.001) and avascular villi (r=-0.348 and p<0.001). Number of syncytial knots correlated positively with, fibrinoid change (r=0.354 and p<0.001), calcification of fibrin (r=0.154 and p<0.02), fibrosis (r= 0.314 and p<0.001) and calcification of the stroma (r=0.282 and p<0.003).

Qualitative changes like endarteritis (r=0.391 and p<0.001) and hypertrophy of the smooth muscles of blood vessels (r=0.233 and p<0.002) correlated positively with the number of syncytial knots.

3. Deposition of Fibrin- Fibrinoid Change

The degree of fibrinoid change did not correlate with gestation (r=-0.036 and p>0.699). Number of syncytial knots had significant association with degree of fibrinoid change (r=0.354 and p<0.001). The degree of fibrinoid change correlated with calcification of fibrin, (r= 0.356 and p<0.001), calcification of stroma (r=0.289 and p<0.020), fibrosis (r=0.289 and p<0.024) and calcified blood vessels (r=0.279 and p<0.003). The degree of fibrinoid change did not correlate with infarction (r=0.167 and p> 0.086), thrombosis (r=-0.056 and p>0.550) and avascular villi (r=-0.099 and p> 0.400).

4. Avascular T.C.V

The degree of avascular terminal villi had significant positive relationship with the amount of stromal tissues (r=0.329 and p<0.002) and villus dimension (r=0.289 and p<0.0026). Avascular terminal villi had significant negative relationship with endarteritis (r=-0.273 and p<0.01), smooth muscle hypertrophy of blood vessels (r=-0.239 and p<0.025), fibrosis (r=-0.333 and p<0.022) and syncytial knots (r=-0.348 and p<0.001).

5. Fibrosis

The degree of fibrosis correlated with syncytial knots (r=0.314 and p<0.001), fibrinoid change (r=0.289 p<0.024), calcification of fibrin, (r=0.239 and p<0.011), calcification of stroma (r=0.497 and p<0.001), endarteritis (r=0.351 and p<0.001), smooth muscle hypertrophy of blood vessels (r=0.303 and p<0.001) and calcified blood vessels (r=0.269 and p<0.004).

Fibrosis correlated negatively with avascular villi (r=-0.333 p<0.022), amount of stroma (r=-0.299 p<0.002) and villous dimension (r=-0.326 p<0.001).

Fibrous tissue formation did not have any relationship with gestational age or blood pressure or P.I.H.

6. Calcification

Calcification correlated with syncytial knots (r=0.282 p<0.003), fibrinoid change (r=0.289 p<0.022), fibrin calcification (r=0.252 p<0.007), fibrosis (r=0.497 p<0.001) and calcification of blood vessels (r=0.545 p<0.001). Calcification correlated with systolic (r=0.225 p<0.017) and diastolic blood pressure (r=0.195 p<0.039) but there was no relationship with gestational age.

7. Infarction

There was no relationship of fibrosis with infarction. All the microscopic features except endarteritis had no relationship with infarction. Even with the endarteritis the association was negative in response (r=-0.148 p<0.033). Both blood pressure and gestational age did not correlate with infarction.

Relationship of Microscopic Features with Clinical Condition

1. Prematurity

The t test analysis for number of syncytial knots when associated with prematurity was significant. The t test of significance (sample =19) for syncytial knots to normal placenta and prematurity was significant. t=-2.105 and P=0.049; Difference of -4 with lower = -8 and upper = -0.01. When analyzed, having removed all antenatal conditions (mainly P.I.H) this relationship was absent. The t test of significance (sample =13) for syncytial knots to normal placenta and prematurity was not significant. t=-1.716 and P= 0.105; Difference of -2.97 with lower = -6.64 and upper = 0.69. The t test analysis for amount of fibrinoid change when associated with prematurity was significant even when abnormal antenatal conditions were excluded. The t test of significance for fibrinoid change of normal placenta and prematurity groups was significant. t= 3.074 and P= 0.004; Difference of 0.91 with lower = 0.31

and upper = 1.51. The significance was apparent when all normal premature infants were examined. The t test of significance for fibrinoid change of normal placenta and prematurity group was significant. t= 4.367 and P= 0.001; Difference of the mean was 1.0 with lower = 0.57 and upper = 1.51.

In other words there was apparent absence of fibrinoid change in placenta of premature infants.

All the microscopic features including fibrinoid change were less apparent in placentae of premature infant. Only syncytial knots were seen in abundance (as a result of their association with P.I.H) but even this was not evident when only normal premature infants were examined. (There were 4 premature infants who were growth retarded).

2. Dysmature Placenta

Morphological features associated with dysmature placentae included 4 with infarction, 3 with fibrosis, 1 with abnormal insertion of cord and membranes, 1 with small peripheral lobule and 6 with inappropriately small placentae.

However, the t tests of significance for number of syncytial knots (more) and fibrinoid change (less) were significantly different. The t test of significance for syncytial knots to normal placenta and dysmature placenta was significant. t= -2.598 and P= 0.026; Difference of the mean was -7.25 with lower = -13.6 and upper = -1.1. The t test of significance for fibrinoid change to normal placenta and dysmature placenta was significant. t= 3.001 and P= 0.018; Difference of the mean was 0.71 with lower = 0.16 and upper = 1.26.

The t test of significance for infarction, fibrosis and calcification to normal placenta and dysmature placenta was not significant. The t test of significance for calcification of the blood vessels to normal placenta and dysmature placenta was significant. t= 5.597 and P= 0.001; Difference of the mean was 0.11 with lower = 0.07 and upper = 0.15.

Incidentally, there was no association with both systolic and diastolic blood pressure.

Calcification was more evident in normal placenta.

3. Low Maternal BMI

There were 23 placentae of mothers with low B.M.I and 18 of them were examined microscopically 5 were with infarction, 2 with fibrosis, 1 with abnormal shape, 2 with abnormal insertion of cord and membranes and 6 placentae were inappropriately small and only 6 placentae did not show macroscopic changes. Altogether 70% of the placentae (16) had morphological abnormalities. 9 mothers out of the 23 had newborns with birth weight below 2500 gm.

Avascular villous (their dimension) significantly associated with placentae of the newborns whose mothers nutrition was poor during pregnancy albeit for their significant reduction in size. The t= 2.431 and P= 0.024; Difference of the mean was 2.3 with lower = 0.33 and upper = 4.3. The t test of significance for infarction to normal placenta and placentae of mother with low maternal BMI (poor nutrition category) placenta was significant. The t= -2.748 and P= 0.012; Difference of the mean was -0.48 with lower = -0.83 and upper = -0.11. The t test of significance for syncytial knots to normal placenta and placentae of mother with low maternal B.M.I was not significant. t= -1.266 and P= 0.215; Difference of the mean was -1.96 with lower = -5.1 and upper = 1.2. The t test of significance for fibrinod change to normal placenta and placentae of mother with low maternal BMI was not significant. t= 1.274 and P= 0.209; Difference of the mean was 0.41 with lower = 0.24 and upper = 1.1. The t test of significance for calcification of the stroma to normal placenta and placentae of mother with low maternal BMI was not significant. t=0.565 and P= 0.580; Difference of the mean was 0.34 with lower = 0.93 and upper = 1.6.

Only two microscopic features were detected significantly.

They were avascular villi (smaller in diameter) and infarction.

Relative lack of fibrinoid change of villi, syncytial knots and calcification of the stroma was seen in placentae of the mothers with low maternal B.M.I and the avasccular villi present were smaller in dimension.

Infarction was seen more often in placenta of mothers with low B.M.I.

4. P.I.H

Systolic blood pressure and diastolic blood pressures correlated with the number of synsytial knots ($r=0.183$ $p<0.006$ and $r=0.146$ and $p<0.030$) respectively. Terminal villous fibrinoid change correlated with diastolic pressure ($r=0.211$ $p<0.024$) but not with systolic pressure ($r=0.135$ and $p>0.149$). The t test of significance for syncytial knots to normal placenta and PIH was significant. $t= -3.411$ $P= 0.001$; Difference of -5 with lower -8 = and upper = -2. Infarction had significant relationship, whereas the fibrosis did not have any relationship with P.I.H. The t test of significance for infarction to normal placenta and P.I.H was significant with $t= -3.526$ $P= 0.001$; Difference of -0.422 with lower = -0.68 and upper = -0.18. The t test of significance for dimensions of fibrinoid villi to normal placenta and P.I.H was significant. $t= 2.252$ and $P= 0.036$; Difference of 4.4 with lower = 0.32 and upper = 8.4. However, the t test of significance for terminal villous fibrin calcification to normal placenta and PIH was not significant. $t= -0.536$ and $P= 0.595$; Difference of -0.19 with lower = -0.95 and upper = 0.54.

Syncytial knots and infarction were present in P.I.H but fibrinoid change was relatively absent.

7. Discussion

1. Defining Growth Restricted Infants

Foetal B.M.I was utilized to define growth restriction. Foetal B.M.I less than 10.5 identified all intra-uterine growth restricted infants above 37 weeks gestation. For infants under 37 weeks of gestation foetal BMI below 10 identified the growth retarded. 11% of the mothers were identified as having intrauterine growth retarded infants (34). In Sri-Lankan context, extremely low or extremely high foetal B.M.I according to gestation needed identification.

Those above or below the defined value should be considered as abnormally grown infants.

2. Defining Poor Maternal Nutrition

Foetal B.M.I was found to be a better index to define growth restriction. Foetal B.M.I two standard deviations according to gestational age were utilized as a retrospective indicator of poor maternal nutrition. The objective was to define nutritionally compromised mothers having excluded all other conditions contributing to IUGR. Additionally a point below 10th centile of the maternal B.M.I at delivery was defined as the cut off point for poor maternal nutrition. The use of B.M.I was not a panacea for inherent problems of analysis of maternal weight but it was used to minimize the effects of height on weight. Maternal B.M.I at early pregnancy was not utilized in defining the cut off point since it was possible for a mother who conceives with a low B.M.I to gain weight and thereby gain adequate B.M.I in latter part of pregnancy.

In the context of defining poor maternal nutrition, maternal BMI below 20 at delivery (prospective) and foetal B.M.I below two standard deviations (retrospective) at birth were useful parameters.

3. Defining Categories of I.U.G.R

Intrauterine growth retardation / restriction was due to many etiologies.

Poor nutrition was only one of them.

Other etiological categories included, P.I.H, congenital abnormalities, multiple pregnancies, maternal heart disease, placental Dysmaturity and unknown and undetermined.

Only 17.5% of infants (6) could be defined as purely nutritionally deficient out of 34 growth retarded infants due to various etiologies. 21% was due to P.I.H (9). 17.5% was due to various maternal (5) and foetal conditions (congenital abnormalities, maternal heart disease and multiple pregnancies). Placental factors (10) determining growth retardation was 29%.

15% was undetermined (4).

In altogether 44% the cause of growth restriction was not detected or determined clinically.

4. Low Birth Weight Infants

Four (4) infants who were above 2500 gm but were growth restricted as defined by foetal B.M.I in this study were not included as growth restricted by Low Birth weight Criterion. Nearly 50% of infants of appropriate foetal B.M.I were included in the Low Birth Weight infants. Premature infants with appropriate foetal B.M.I for gestation but below 2500 gm would be grouped together as Low Birth Weight if WHO criterion was to be utilized.

4 premature infants were defined as growth restricted in the present study. Lumping premature infants, into low birth weight category without qualification for gestation was fraught with inaccuracy as far as the foetal growth restriction was concerned.

WHO Low Birth Weight (LBW) criterion inappropriately increased the percentage of so called Low Birth Weight infants to 18%. For no obvious scientific reason over 7% of the infants were considered to be born to mothers who were under nourished.

The arbitrary definition of maternal nutrition as a cause of I.U.G.R was a serious impediment to study of foetal growth, especially growth retarded newborns in Sri-Lankan context.

Placental Morphological Findings

This study was instigated to define normal placental features so that abnormality could be defined without subjective bias. Histoplathological features such as calcification, syncytial knots, fibrin deposition, infarction, fibrosis and avascular villi had significant expression in the placenta during pregnancy.

Villous Dimensions

For analytical purposes the villi with 4 to 6 blood vessels were considered representative. There was significant increase in connective tissue (stroma) elements and villous dimensions from 36 weeks to 40 weeks of gestation, in those villi with 4 to 6 blood vessels. There is no reason why the stromal tissue should stop growing in normally functioning placenta and that was what was observed in this study. The lack of appropriate growth up to 40 weeks of gestation may be a sign of placental compromise. However, there was no change in dimensions of terminal villi with 4 to 6 blood vessels in various antenatal conditions including P.I.H. In large placentae and in anaemic mothers the villous dimensions were comparatively larger, possibly due to congestion / vasodilatation but the numbers were not sufficient to evaluate the statistical significance.

Microscopic Entities and their associations and relationships

1. Amount of Villus Stroma

The amount of villus stroma per high power field showed an increase with advancing gestation up to 40 weeks, contrary to the accepted norm. There was notable negative correlation of amount of stromal tissues to syncytial knots, terminal villous fibrinoid change, calcification of fibrin and fibrosis. It appears the amount of stromal tisuue is related to the vascularity of the planeta. The villous dimension diminishes in size when there are associated conditions that compromises the vascularity of the placenta.

2. Syncytial Knots

The number of syncytial knots per high power field did not show any increase with advancing gestation contrary to the accepted norm. Though, an unexpected finding, the number of syncytial knots per high power field did not increase with the gestation from 36 up to 40 weeks. However the number increased significantly with blood pressure (P.I.H) irrespective of the gestational age. Increase in number of syncytial knots indicated the foetal response to maternal P.I.H and its relationship with gestation was probably coincidental.

However, increased number of syncytial knots were consistently and significantly associated with both abnormal maternal (P.I.H), foetal (I.U.G.R) and pathological (Dysmature placentae) conditions.

A notable lack of relationship with syncytial knots was seen with mothers with poor nutrition and normal premature infants.

3. Deposition of Fibrin like Material- Fibrinoid Change

Even though, fibrinoid change was not seen significantly in P.I.H, there was an association of fibrinoid change with diastolic blood pressure and increased syncytial knots. The arguments for the view that the fibrinoid change is a pathological entity are the positive relationship with syncytial knots, fibrosis and calcification of the stroma and the negative relationship with amount of stromal tissue and villous dimension.

It may be that it starts with subtle injury and that it changes its course depending on the associated clinical condition. Its relative absence in premature infants and progressive accumulation in mature infants and the lack of relationship with avascular villi further supports this view.

In this regard the fibrinoid change can be taken as a satisfactory indirect indicator of vascular injury.

Deposition of fibrin like material and their eventual calcification probably indicate subtle injury that causes leakage of this material from injured blood vessels.

Association of fibrinoid change with diastolic blood pressure, syncytial knots and fibrosis are valid indicators of their origin as a result of vascular injury.

It is difficult to discern whether the fibrinoid change is physiological or pathological if analyzed in isolation. Similarly arguments could be put forward for the view that fibrinoid change is physiological.

Probably it is not pathological as shown by its relative absence in P.I.H and Dymature placenta. Its relative lack of presence in placenta of poorly nourished mothers can be another reasons to support fibrinoid change as physiological.

Its relative lack of presence (minimal) in placenta of normal premature infants is difficult to explain unless it is explained that fibrinoid change as an event in maturation.

However, the fibrinoid change did not change with gestation to support this view. But if it is proposed that that fibrinoid material is eventually changed to avacular hyalinized component as it is formed, we can explain the lack of relationship with gestation.

Its association with diastolic blood pressure and its relative absence with P.I.H is a serious stumbling block to this argument and it appears vascular injury promotes its formation.

Only 9 (25%) out of 36 infants whose mother had P.I.H had significant growth restriction.

It is apparent, most of the mothers with P.I.H escape any injury to placenta and its blood vessels. On that ground we can discount the lack of relationship of fibrinoid change with P.I.H.

Whether it is physiological or pathological, its evolution is dynamic and does not remain static and is either removed or converted to avacular tissue or forms the framework for formation or invasion of new blood vessels.

It may be that proper nutrition is necessary for its formation.

They are formed both from maternal and foetal components.

It can be argued that fibrinoid material may be formed, whatever its origin or ts cause, in the first instance and it may provide as a framework for vascularization of the rapidly growing and maturing placenta, in the second half of the pregnancy.

In that context one has to assume it is a dynamic process and not static element.

Even though, there is some increase in amount fibrinoid material in the placenta of mature infants this increase was statistically not significant as far as the advancing gestational age is concerned. If that is the case it may not point to maturation of the placenta. However, the lack of relationship with gestation may be due to its subsequent conversion to avascular tissue or mature connective tissue.

It may be a stage before formation avascular terminal villous elements or mature vascularized connective tissue with advancing gestation.

The masking effect of its relationship to gestation could be due to its latter conversion to either avascular tissue or mature choroidal tissue. The avid staining reaction of fibrinod like material as opposed to hyaline like appearance of avascular villous tissue may be relevant.

When formed fibrinoid material probably has an open protein structure that gives it an avid reaction with staining.

Its relationship may be similar to fibronectin in healing and repair process. Epithelialization by syncytiocytoblast epithelial elements probably makes it to mature and become hyalinized.

It may even subsequently become vascularized.

If fibrinod material is not pathological, the sequence of events that follows is fibrinod change, epithelilization, hyalinization, avascular tissue formation and finally vascularization to mature connective tissue containing blood vessels.

Fibrinod material may even be a grand decoy with an evolutionary bluff in mind. It has maternal elements with potential antigenic material to elicit foetal response. Equally it has foetal elements that have potentiality to produce maternal reaction. The two elements maternal and foetal in combination especially when not fully epitheliazied by syncytiotrophoblast probably fool the immuno-potent cells to accept them as self until open protein structure with antigenic determinants are cleverly hidden as hyaline material in avascular villous elements.

It is better for it to be ***left as an unknown entity*** and its frequent accompaniment in the latter half pregnancy warrants careful delineation of associated factors including gestational age.

In whatever, context whether physiological or pathological fibrinoid change is a placental mystery that needs proper prospective study.

4. Avascular Terminal Villi

The presence of avascular villi seems to be a function of growth of the villi and did not indicate vascular occlusion of preformed blood vessels. It seemed that the stromal tissue was accommodated without blood vessels. Furthermore, the avascular terminal villi were not significantly associated with increase in systolic blood pressure. Avascularization of terminal villi was not a pathological response to systolic or diastolic stress.

It could be expressed as an index of villus or placental maturity with gestation. Increase in the formation of avascular villi was observed with advancing gestation in the normal placentae as well as abnormal placentae. There was positive relationship with stromal elements (which also showed an increase in amount up to 40 week in normal placenta) and negative relationship with number of synsytial knots. In other words presence of syncytial knots was not conducive for the formation of avascular villi. Unlike the number of sysncytil knots that showed direct relationship blood pressure avascular villi did not have any relationship with blood pressure. Avascular villi showed negative relationship with endarteritis and hypertrophy of smooth muscles which had significant relationship positively with syncytial knots. Latter relationships are expressions of vascular changes with high blood pressure (P.I.H). These findings are relevant since formation of avascular villi may be a physiological process that probably indicated aging process of the placenta.

Unlike the increase in stromal tissue (does not occur in abnormal placenta) that occur only in normal placenta, avascular changes of villi can occur irrespective of whether the placentae were normal or abnormal with associated pathological features.

The above observation is relevant, if it is assumed that the fibrinoid change is a pathological entity but it is eventually converted to avascular tissue to avoid potential antigenic stimulation by foetal or maternal immuno-potent cells.

The lack of relationship to blood pressure is suggestive that the formation of avascular villi is probably not related to vascular injury but relatively independent placental event.

Whereas fibrinoid change associated positively with fibrosis, the avacular villi had negative relationship with fibrosis further indicating that it is not a vascular injury but a curious accompaniment of advancing gestation.

In other words when syncytial knots and fibrosis were present the avascular terminal villi were noted for their absence.

Fibrinoid change of villi and syncytial knots indicated vascular injury whereas avascular villi did not.

It may be that in the latter part of pregnancy the blood vessel formation seemed to lag behind the stromal tissue proliferation and not due to obliteration of already established blood vessels.

In some way avascular elements seem to indicate the maturity of the placenta. Further study of this histological feature (curiosity) is indicated.

Aetiology of avascular villous formation is ill defined but probably related to the maturity of the placenta.

Since the use of syncytial knots cannot be used as an indicator of maturation of the placenta in our infants (it is disputed), the use of these elements to assess the maturity of the placenta in relation to gestation is indicated until substantial validity is established in further studies to determine the association of syncytial knots with gestation. The relative smaller size of avascular villous elements in mothers with low maternal BMI probably indicated that adequate nutrition is necessary for their formation.

Formation avascular villous elements may be a stage prior to vascularization (not after) and their formation may be a prerequisite for vascularization.

The assumption here is that the vascularization lags behind the stromal tissue growth. The conversion of fibrinoid materail to avascular tissue can be another assumption.

5. Fibrosis

Fibrosis occurs in placenta as a result of injury. Fibrosis had significant relationship with number of syncytil knots, fibrinoid change, calcification of the fibrinoid, calcification of the stroma, endateritis and hypertrophy of the smooth muscles of the placental blood vessels.

Fibrous tissue formation did not have any relationship with gestational age and blood pressure.

There was no relationship of fibrosis with infarction.

Aetiology of fibrosis was probably multi-faceted. Injuries in early pregnancy do not elicit inflammatory responses due to lack of inflammatory cells but the ultimate placental response to injury is fibrous tissue reaction.

In foetal development, early injury to placenta results in fibrosis whether the injury is result of mechanical injury or infectious or otherwise. It was possible that these injuries were clinically silent but were long standing early injuries.

Fibrosis indicated a result of some old injury but tends to be non progressive. Fibrosis could have been due to many aetiological factors which probably had transient influence on the growth of the placenta.

6. Infarction

There was significant association of infarction with P.I.H, Dysmature placentae and to some degree in maternal poor nutrition. Infarction was not seen when placentae were large as in anaemia and diabetes mellitus where the blood vessels were apparently dilated compared to normal placentae. Infarction indicated vascular compromise and seemed to be progressive especially in P.I.H.

7. Calcification

Calcification had significant associations with the number of syncytial knots, fibrinoid change, calcification of fibrinoid and fibrosis. However, infarction did not associate with calcification. Calcification was seen significantly with increase in blood pressure both systolic and diastolic.

Why calcification occurs in placentas is ill understood.

It is unarguably an end stage of vascular and / or villous tissue injury.

It may be that, most of the injuries to the placenta follow a histologically recognizable patten and sequence.

It starts with formation of syncytial knots (initial reaction to stress), formation fibrinoid material (progressive injury) and calcification of fibrin (end stage of injury), like material with or without fibrous reaction.

Calcification seems to be the final end product in choroidal tissue injury that has not resulted in fibrosis or before the fibrous tissue reaction could ensue. On the other hand calcification may be coincidental with the injuries that occur in placental tissue. Wherever its cause calcification is evidently seen in placenta both in macroscopic and in microscopic examination but because of universal presence its significance has been ignored and underscored.

Qualitative Features

Qualitative features of blood vessels which included endarteritis, calcification, smooth muscle hypertrophy and thrombosis were identified. Isolated histopathological features which included infarctions, fibrosis, oedema, congestion of blood vessels and the evidence of infections which were either focal or diffuse were also noted in the detailed examination of the placentae.

These qualitative features especially calcification, endarteritis and smooth muscle hypertrophy had significant relationship with the quantitatively assessed features.

The progression of pathological events from syncytial knots, to fibrinoid change to calcification to calcification of blood vessels and endarteritis and fibrosis could be assessed, if these features are objectively studied but not in isolation as it is the generally done in routine microscopic examination.

This study was a departure from that tradition.

Associations of Microscopic Features with Clinical entities

1. Findings in PIH

Except fibrosis all other pathological features were significantly associated with P.I.H. They included calcification, infarction and increased syncytial knots.

When associated with I.U.G.R these finding were remarkably intense.

2. Findings in Low Maternal BMI

Significant microscopic features were not detected microscopically in mothers with very low B.M.I. Apart from increased incidence of infarction the other major finding was Low Placental Weight.

The presence of increased number of syncytial knots may exclude nutrition as a cause and look for other aetiological factors was warranted.

Avascular tisuue elements were significantly smaller in size when the maternal BMI was low.

3. Findings in Dysmature Placenta

Significant microscopic features were detected microscopically in Dysmature placentae associated with I.U.G.R. Dysmature placentae were associated with increase in number of syncytial knots and infarction and not with fibrosis, calcification and avascular villi.

The association of fibrinoid change was similar to PIH but was less in degree in Dysmature placentae.

The aietiology of the I.U.G.R in these infants associated with dysmature and abnormal placentae was different from that of P.I.H and poor maternal nutrition. They may be related to the idiopathic intrauterine retardation as described by Salafia.

Further study of this category is warranted.

Findings of Dysmature placenta in this study need refining. in a future study.

4. Findings in Premature Infants

It is apparent when there are no clinical entities the premature infants show histopathological changes similar to placentae of mature infants except the presence of number of syncytial knots (which were less in number) and fibrinoid change. But when infants were affected by P.I.H and I.U.G.R, the placentae of premature infants showed most of the morphological changes except perhaps fibrinoid change. However, the number of premature infants studied was relatively few to make conclusive deductions but the tendencies shown above are clinically relevant.

8. Conclusions

A. Validity of Foetal and Maternal BMI

The conclusions that can be derived form analysis of foetal BMI and maternal BMI are as follows.

10th centile for BMI in the second half of pregnancy was a useful indicator that defined nutritionally compromised mothers. 45% of these mothers under B.M.I below 20 had born newborns below 2500 gm and 60% of them had placental abnormalities. The normal range for B.M.I of our mothers was 20 to 29. Further increase of B.M.I above 29 did not enhance the foetal growth significantly.

Foetal B.M.I 2 SD below the mean (B.M.I 10 for premature infants and 10.5 for mature infants) was a reliable indicator of growth restriction of our infants and retrospectively determined the poor maternal nutrition (provided that other clinical conditions that caused I.U.G.R were excluded).

B. Validity of Histopathological Entities

Several conclusions could be made at the end of histological and histopathological examinations.

1. The microscopic examination of the placenta was useful in determining features that were associated with clinical, pathological (P.I.H, Maternal Low B.M.I, placental Dysmaturity) as well as growth restricted infants.

2. There was ***broad agreement*** with the histological features described internationally but there were also ***significant departures*** from international findings.

The histopathological findings observed in broad agreement with international findings were fibrosis, infarction and calcification.

They were seen in P.I.H and placentae of growth retarded infants.

3. In contrast to international observations the increase in number of syncytial knots and the reduction in stromal tissue with increase in maturation of the placenta were not observed in this study.

Observations made in this study were objective but not subjective unlike some of the international interpretations.

4. An assessment of the amount of stromal tissue in terminal villi with four blood vessels showed significant increase of stromal tissue elements up to 40 weeks of gestation.

5. Whereas the syncytial knots did not increase with gestation.

6. However, syncytial knots ***increased with both systolic and diastolic blood pressure.***

7. There was association of syncytial knots with growth restriction of the infants except with growth restriction due to poor maternal nutrition.

8. The presence of syncytial knots indicated some sort of stress to the growing placenta and foetus.

9. Additionally, syncytial knots were remarkably absent in placenta of nutritionally deficient mothers.

Their presence was a strong indication for looking for causes other than nutrition for growth retardation.

10. Aetiology of avascular villous formation is ill defined but probably related to the maturity of the placenta. Since the use of syncytial knots for our infants is disputed, the use of these elements to assess the maturity of the placenta in relation to gestation is indicated (until substantial validity is established in further studies to determine the association of syncytial knots with gestation).

11. It is difficult to discern whether the fibrinoid change is physiological or pathological if analyzed in isolation. Probably it is not pathological in some instances and pathological in others.

Associated conditions determine whether the fibrinoid material is normal or abnormal.

12. Why calcification occurs in placentas is ill understood. It is unarguably an end stage of vascular and / or villous tissue injury.

Calcification seems to be the final end point of injury or may be coincidental.

13. Infarction indicated vascular compromise and seemed to be progressive especially in P.I.H.

14. Aetiology of fibrosis was ill defined.
Even though there was some association with P.I.H it was probably not in relation to blood pressure but due to some other factor or factors independent of P.I.H.

15. *Findings of Dysmature placenta in this study need further refining.*
Aietiology of these newborns with I.U.G.R associated with abnormal placentae was different from that of P.I.H and poor nutrition.

16. Premature infants showed significant pathological changes and nearly 30% of them were associated with P.I.H.
The apparent increase in number of syncytial knots was related to the associated P.I.H in our newborns.

In normal premature newborns there was no significant increase in pathological events that included syncytial knots.

There was also apparent lack of fibrinoid change in premature infants.

17. Qualitative features of microscopic examination had associations with histological and histopathological features defined in this study. These qualitative features especially calcification, endarteritis and smooth muscle hypertrophy of the blood vessels had significant relationship with the quantitatively assessed features.

18. The progression of pathological events from fibrinoid change to syncytial knots, to calcification, to calcification of blood vessels and endarteritis and fibrosis are very poorly defined in pathological and clinical context.

It is difficult to define the sequence of events, since these features seen under the microscope cannot be objectively followed.

The closest approximation to objective study is to define inter-category relationships of these features and study them in somewhat objective manner, not in isolation but as a part of the overall or global picture. that may emerge.

Then, the routine microscopic examination becomes a valid tool in pathological context.

This study was a departure from the normal tradition of descriptive nature, often tagged with presumptive but not very well substantiated clinical judgment.

Both *quantitative* and *qualitative* features were analyzed to bring some objectivity to the examination of the placenta at the time of delivery.

Future Studies

Statistically significant numbers were not available for prematurity (for each gestational age category), diabetes mellitus, anaemia and other antenatal conditions.

It is proposed that future studies should concentrate and evaluate them.

Chart 1

Figure 3.1. Relationship of Antenatal Maternal Weights to Gestational Age in days

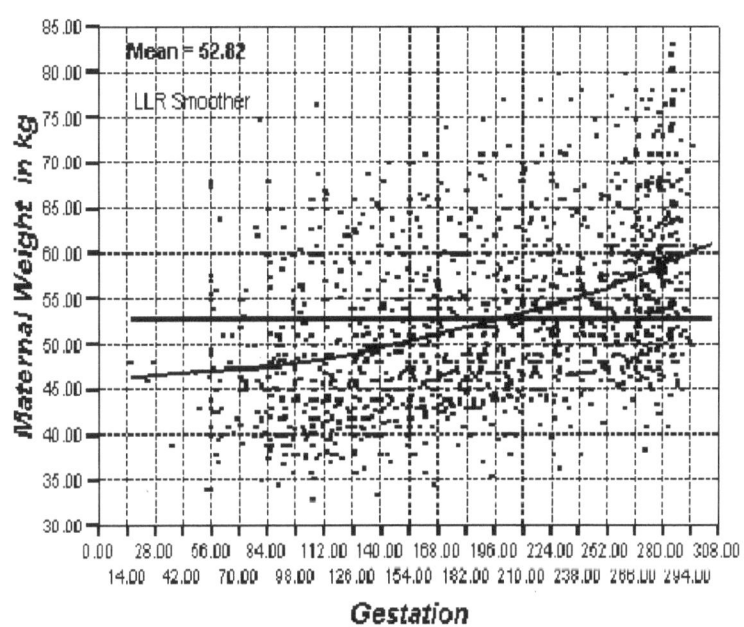

Chart 1

Chart2

Figure 3.2. Relationship of Antenatal Maternal Weights to Gestational Age in weeks

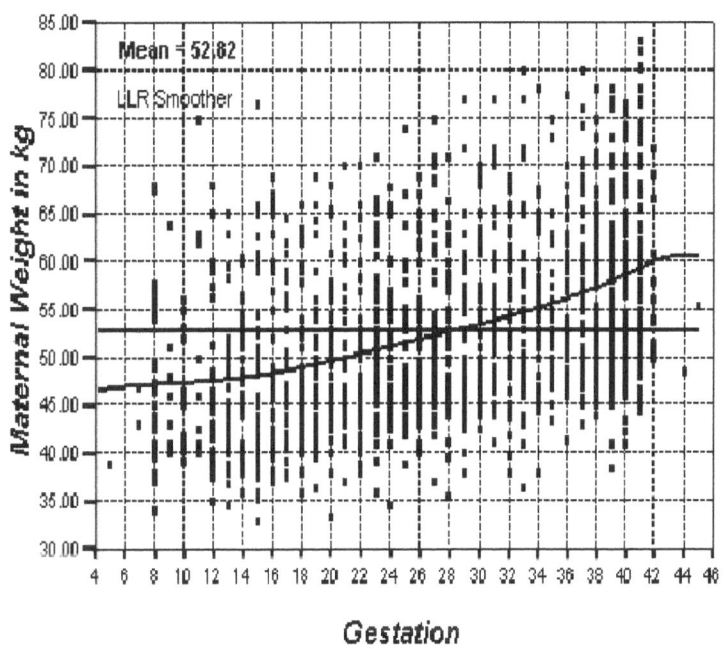

Chart 2

64

Chart 3

Figure 3.3. Relationship of Gestational Age (in weeks) to Maternal BMI

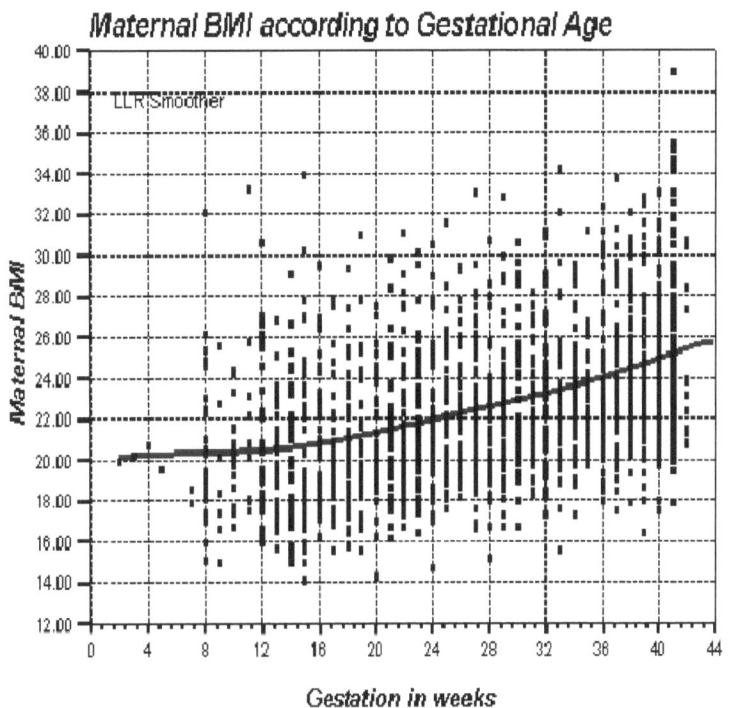

Chart 3

Chart 4

Figure 3.4. Relationship of Gestational Age (in days) to Maternal BMI

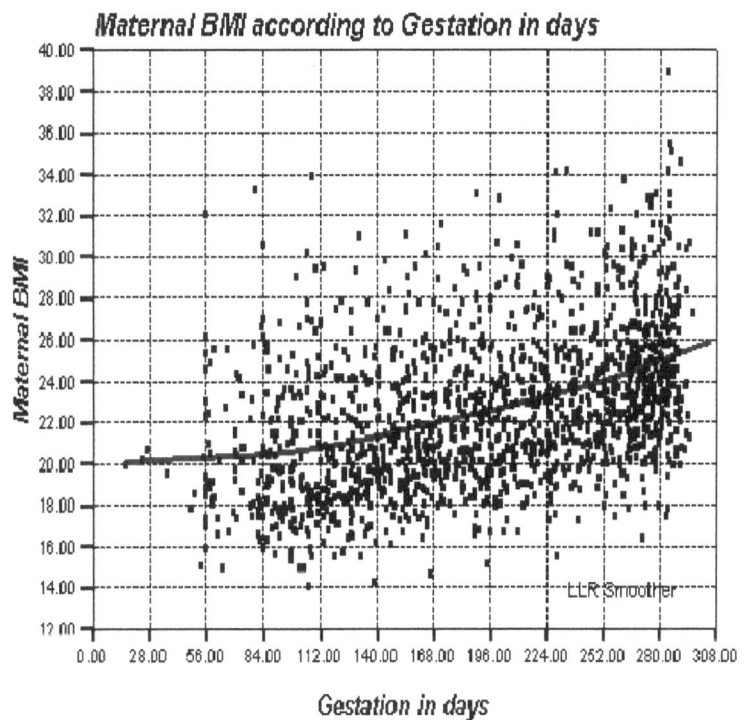

Chart 4

68

Chart 5

Figure 3.5. Relationship of Gestational Age (95% CI) to Maternal BMI

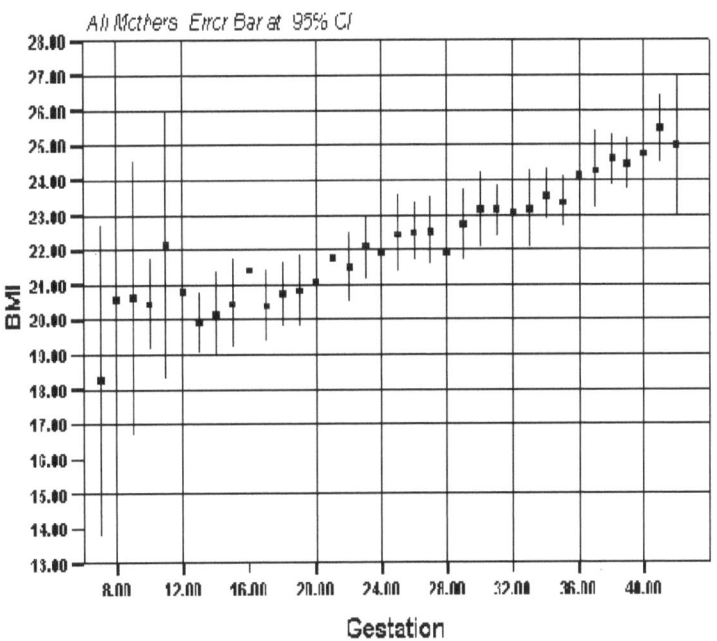

Chart 5

70

Chart 6

Figure 3. 6. Relationship of Placental Weight to Maternal BMI

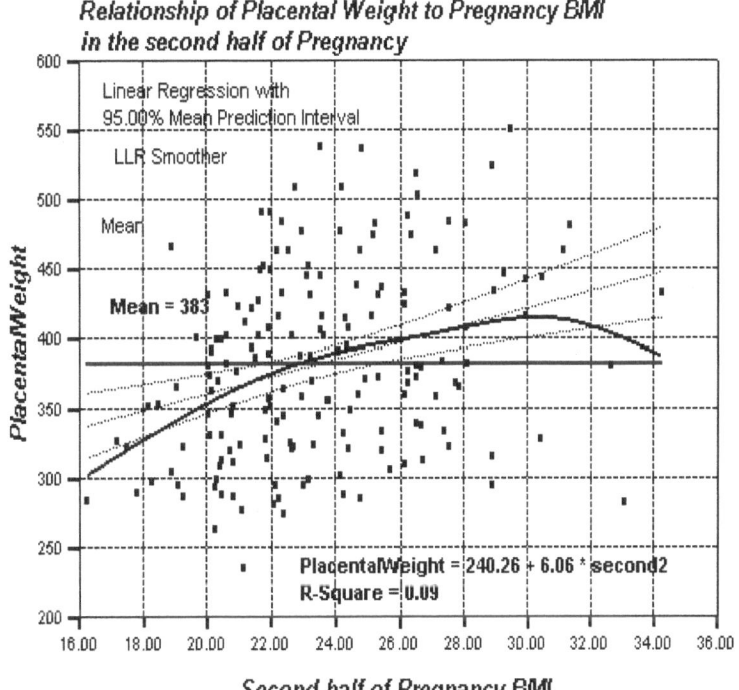

Chart 6

Chart 7

Figure 3.7. Percentile Chart for Maternal BMI (32 t0 42 weeks)

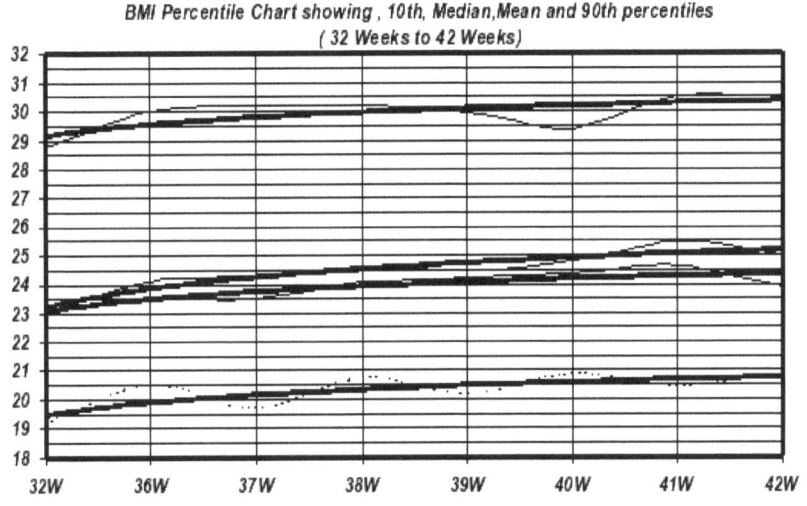

Chart 7

Chart 8

Figure 3.8. Percentile Chart for Maternal BMI (32 to 42 weeks)

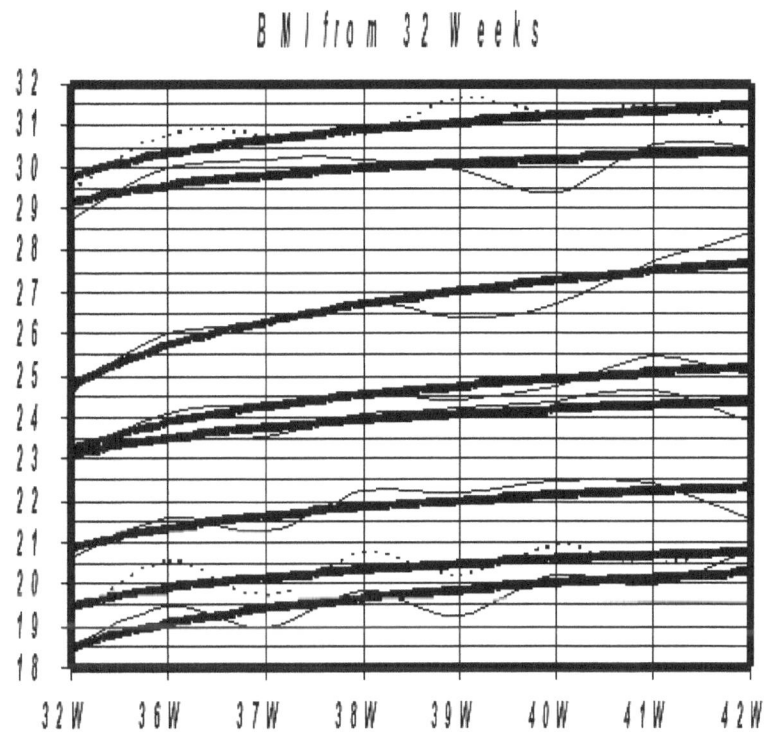

Chart 8

Chart 9

Figure 3.9. Relationship of Maternal BMI at Delivery to Birth Weight

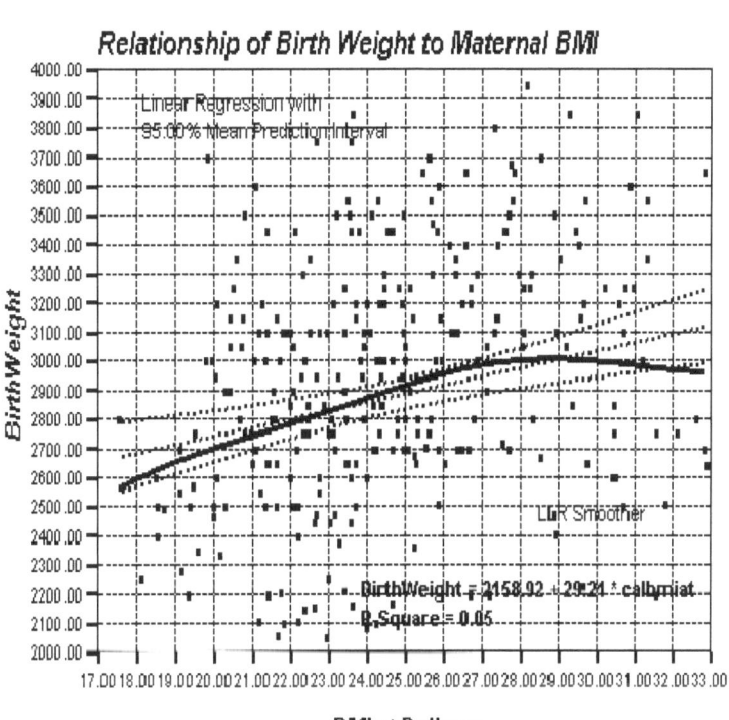

Chart 9

Chart 10

Figure 3.10. Relationship of Maternal BMI at Delivery to Foetal BMI

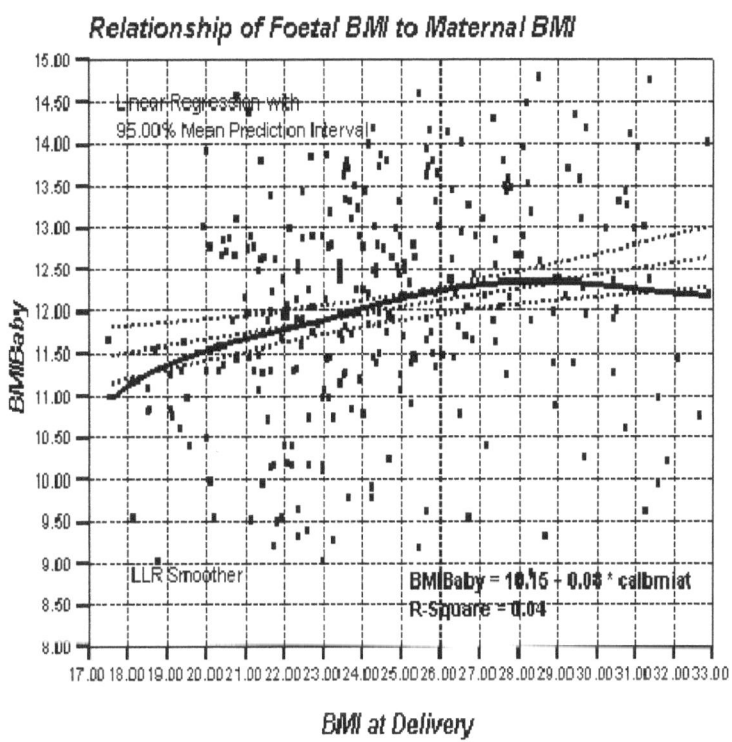

Chart 10

80

Chart 11

Figure 3.2. Relationship of Foetal BMI to Gestation in weeks

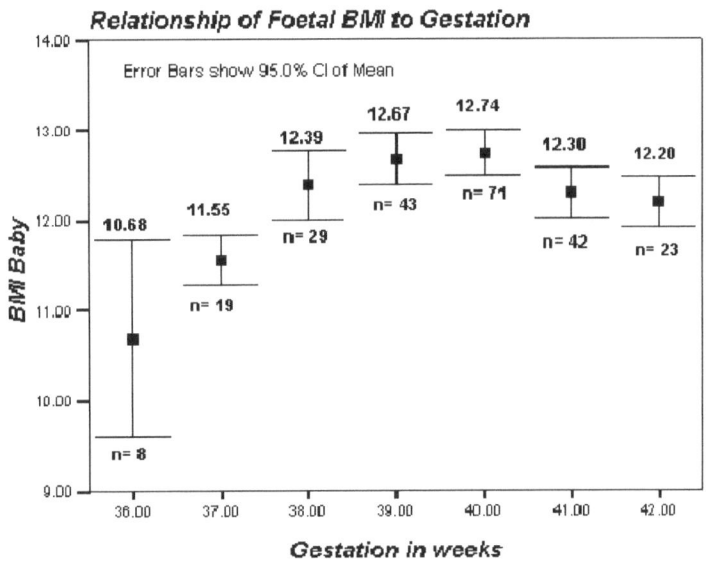

Figure 3.1. Relationship of Foetal BMI to Gestational Age

Chart 11

Chart 12

Figure 3.2. Relationship of Foetal BMI to Placental Weight (Infants with Appropriate Foetal BMI)

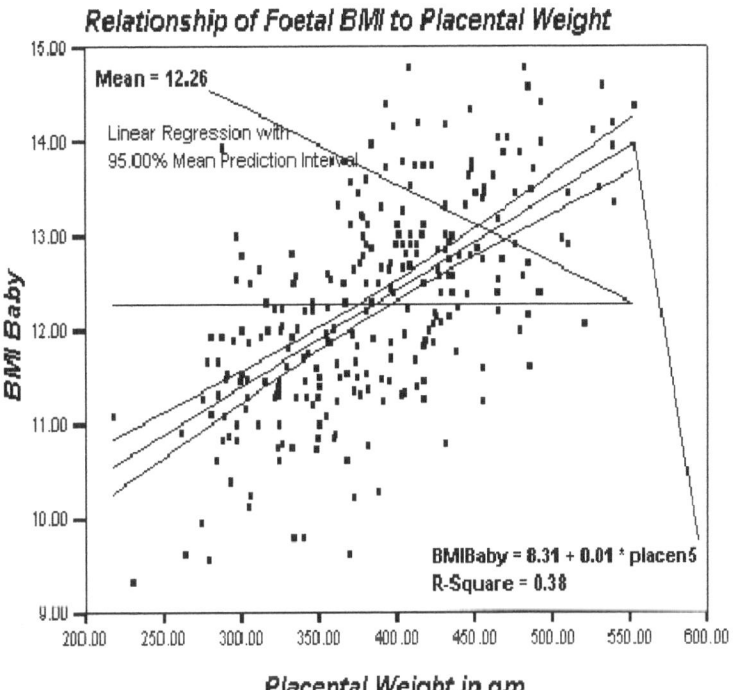

Chart 12

Chart 13
Avacular Villi

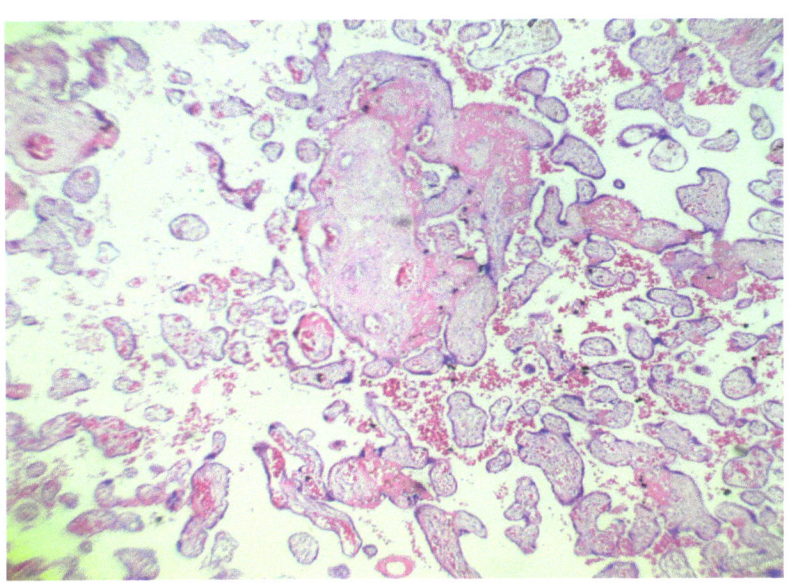

Image 1

86

Chart 14
Fibrinoid Villi

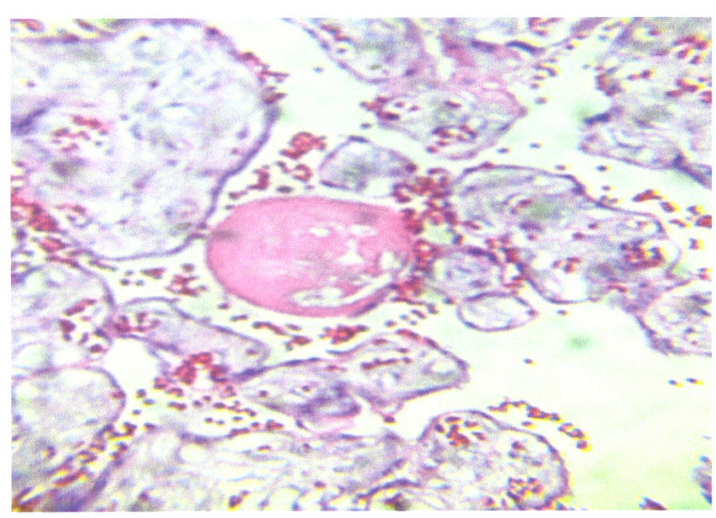

Image 2

88

Chart 15
Calcification

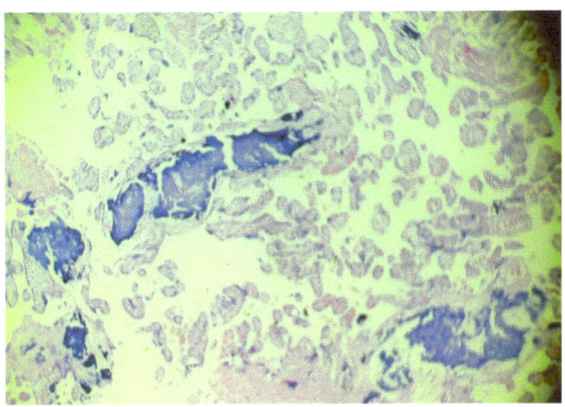

Image 3

Chart 16
Endarteritis

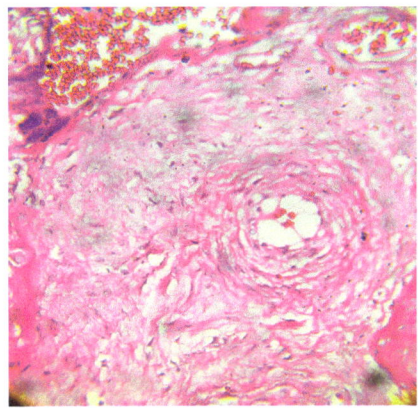

Image 4

Chart 17
Syncytial knots

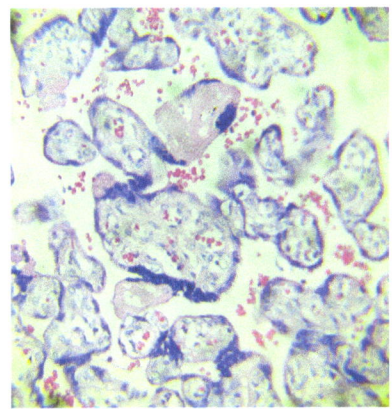

Image 5

Chart 18

Villi

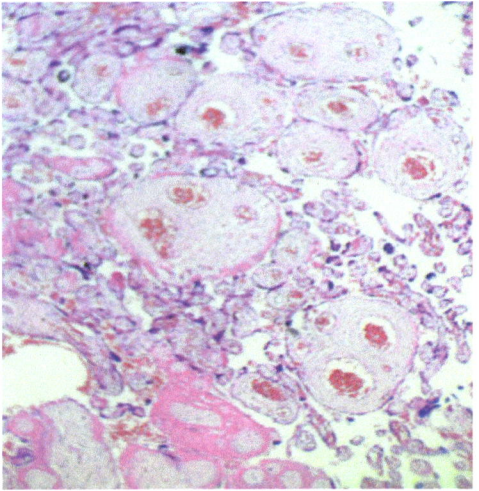

Image 6

Chart 19
Villi

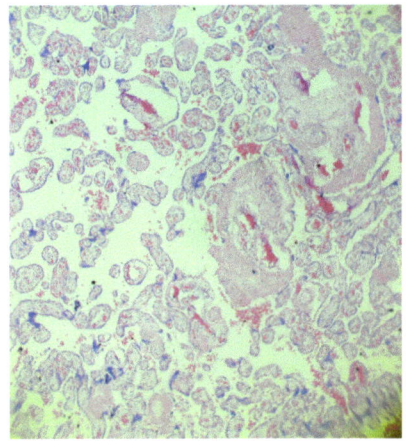

Image 7

98

Chart 20

Stem Villi

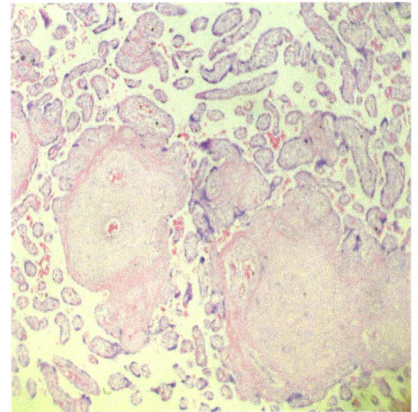

Image 8

100

Chart 21

Fibrosis

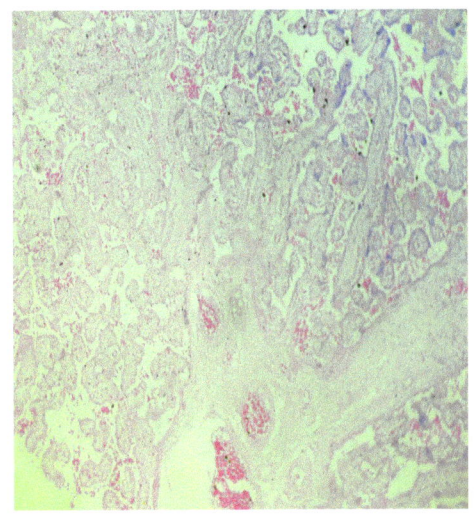

Image 9

Chart 22
Terminal Chorionic Villi

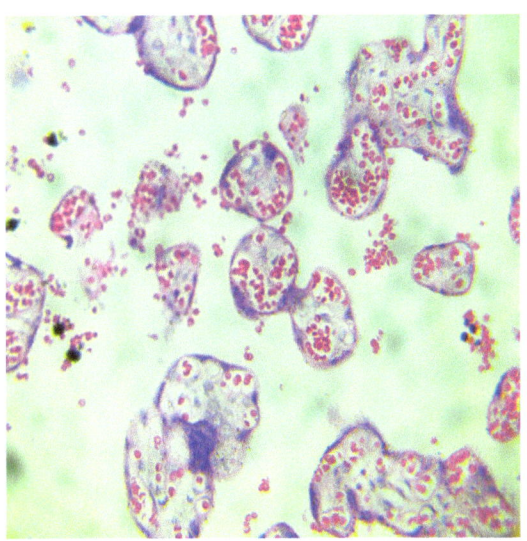

Image10

References

1. Abrams BF, Laros RK: Pregnancy weight, weight gain and birth weight: Amer J of Obstect and Gynae: 15,503-509, 1986

2. Adair FL, Thelander H: A study of the weight and dimensions of the placenta and its relation to birth weight of the newborn infant: Am J Obstet Gynecol 10: 172, 1925

3. Allen AH: Recent developments in maternal nutrition and their implication for practitioners: American J Clinical Nutrition 59 (2) suppli: 439-541, 1994

4. Battaglia FC, Lubchenco LO: A practical classification of newborn infants by weight and gestational age: J Pediatrics: 71: 2,159-163, 1967

5. Barasi M.E; 1997

6. Barker DJP, Osmond C: Infant mortality, childhood nutrition and ischaemic heart disease in England and Wales: Lancet: 1077-1081.1986

7. Barker DJP, Osmond C, Winter PD et al: Weight in infancy and death from ischaemic heart disease; Lancet: ii: 577-580, 1989

8. Barker DJP, Bull AR, Osmond C, Simmonds SJ: Foetal and placental size and risk of hypertension in adult life: BMJ: 301: 259-259-262, 1990

9. Battaglia FC, Lubchenco LO: A practical classification of newborn infants by weight and gestational age: J Pediatrics: 71: 2,159-163, 1967

10. Beconsfield P, Villee C: Placenta: A Neglected Experimental Animal: Elmsford NY Pergamon Press Inc, 1979.

11. Beconsfield P, Birdwood G, Beconsfield R: The Placenta; Scientific American, 80-89, 1996

12. Bernirschke K: The placenta in the context of history and modern medical practice: Arch Pathol Lab Med: 115,663-667, 1991.

13. Benirschke K, Kaufmann P. Pathology of Human Placenta. Comparison of Published cord lengths: 2nd Edition New York NY Springer Verlag NY Inc; 1990, 1995

14. Billewitz WZ, Kemsley WFF, Thomson AM: Brit J Prev Soc Med: 16, 183, 1962

15. Brosens I, Dixon HG and Robertson W.B, 1977

16. Brown JE Abrams BF Lederman SA, Naeye RL, Rees JM, Taffel S, et all; 1990

17. Collan Y; Reproducibility, neglected cornerstone of medical diagnosis. In Collan Y, Romppanen T, eds. Morphometry in Morphological diagnosis. Kuopio: Kuopio University Press, 1982

18. Dissanayake SBA.; Maternal Parameters associated with Birth Weight and Placental Weight in Sri-Lankan mothers, 2004

19. Dissanayake SBA; Development of Antenatal Chart for Maternal BMI; 2005

20. Eastmen NJ and Jacson EC: The bearing on maternal weight gain and pre-pregnancy weight on birth weight and full term pregnancies: Obstect Gynarcol Surv: 23:1003-25, 1968

21. Emanuel RI, Robinson BG, Seely EW, et al. Coirticotrophin releasing hormone lkeels in human plasma and amniotic fluid during gestation. Cli Endocrinol: 40:257-62, 1994

22. Gardorsi J, Chang A, Kalyan B, Sahota D Symmonds EN: Customized antenatal growth charts: Lancet: 339:283-7, 1992

23. Gruenwald P, Hoang Ngoc Minh: Evaluation of organ and body weights in perinatal pathology: Ame J Obst & Gynae: 82: 2: 312-319, 1961

24. Gruenwald P: The Placenta and its maternal supply line. Lancaster Pennsylvania, Medical and Teaching Publishing, 1975, pp 1-17

25. Hoffmann HJ; 1974,, Kramer MS; 1987

26. Kliman HJ, The Placenta Revealed; Am J Pathol: 143:332-6, 1994

27. Kliman HJ, Perrotta PL, Jones DC: The efficacy of Placental Biopsy; Am J Obstet Gynecol: 173:1084-8, 1995

28. Kramer MS; 1987

29. Langston.C, C.Kaplan, T.Macpherson, E.Manci, K.Peevy, B.Clark, C.Murtagh et al.1997.Practice guide line for examination of the placenta.121:449-476.

30. Lindsay RS, Lindsay RM, Edwards CRW et al Inhibition of 11β hydroxylated dehydrogenase in in pregnant rats and anf the programming of blood pressure in offspring. Hypertension; 27:1200-4; 1996

31. Lingley-Evans SC Phillips GJ Benedicktsson R et al; Protein intake in Pregnancy, placental glucocorticoid metabolism and the programming of hypertension. Placenta; 17:167-72; 1996

32. Lissauer T and Clayden, G, 2007

33. Lubchenco LO, Hansma n C, Dressler M Boyd F Intrauterine growth as estimated from liveborn birth weght data at 24 to 42 weeks of gestaton:Pediatrics:32:793, 1963

34. Lubchenco L, Why choose three weeks on one side of the peak incidence (40 weeks) and two weeks on the other side, unless to avoid observation of moderate risk infants? Care of the high risk Neonate Cha 4 -p 67; 1979

35. Naeye.R.L.and N.Tafari.1983.Risk Factors in Pregnancy and Disease of the Foetus and Newborn. Baltimore: Williams & Wilkins.22-23.

36. Naeye R.I. Do placental weights have clinical significance? Hum Pathol 18:387-391, 1987

37. Naeye RL: Maternal body weight and pregnancy outcome: American Journal of Clinical Nutrition; 52:273-279; 1990

38. McCormick MC; 1986

39. Rayburn W, Sander C: Histopathological examination of the placenta in chronic growth retarded foetus, Am J Perinatol, 1989

40. Roertson WB, Bronsen I, Dixon HG, The pathological response of the vessels of the placental bed to hypertensive pregnancy: Pathol Bacteriol: 93:581-592,1967

41. Salafia CM, Vintzileousw AW: Why all placentas should be examined by a Pathologist in 1990: Am J Obstect Gynecol: 163:1282-93, 1990

42. Salafia CM, Minior VK, Perrullo JC et al

43. Sciscione A.C, Gorman R, Callan N.A. Adjustment of birth weight standards for maternal and infant characteristics improves the prediction of outcome in the small for gestational age infant. Am. J. Obstect & Gynec; 17:544-547,1996

44. Thompson (1968) et al

45. Van den Berg JB, Yerushalmy J: Birth weight and gestation as indices of immaturity: Am J Dis Child.J Pediatrics: 109:43, 1965

46. Van den Berg B, Yerushalmy J. The relationship of the rate of intrauterine growth of infants of low birth weight to mortality, morbidity and congenital abnormalities. J.PEDIATRICS; 69:4:531-545,1967

47. Winick M, Noble A; Quantative changes in DNA, RNA and protein during prenatal and post natal growth in the rat: Developmental Biology: 12,451, 1965

48. Winick M, Noble A; Quantitative changes in ribonucleic acids and protein during normal growth of rat placenta: Nature 212: 34, 1966

49. Winick M, Noble A; Cellular response in rats during malnutrition at various stages: J. Nutr: 89:300, 1966

50. Winick M, Coscia A, Noble A: Cellular growth in human placenta. I Normal Placental Growth: Pediatrics 39: 2,248, 1967

51. Winick M, Noble A: Cellular response with increased feeding of neonatal rats: J. Nutr: 91:179, 1967

Appendix I

Microscopic Measurement

Method of measurement of an object by means of a microscope involves the use of a Stage Micrometer and an Eye-piece Micrometer of which there are various types for various purposes.

Stage Micrometer (SM)

Stage Micrometer consists of a glass slide with a linear millimeter scale engraved upon it. The scale has one hundred 0.01 mm (1 µm) divisions, every 10 divisions being marked by extended lines. The engraved portion is protected by a cover slip.

Eye-piece Micrometer (graticule) or scale (EM)

It consists of a glass disc usually 21mm in diameter. On its surface is an engraved linear scale with one hundred equal divisions; every tenth division being numbered and indicated by a longer line. This scale is 1 cm in length. The size of the divisions is arbitrary.

Calibration of eye-piece scale or graticule

The eye-piece graticule must be calibrated at a given tube length for each combination of ocular and objective. If any one factor is changed the graticule must be re-calibrated. To calibrate the eye-piece graticule the stage micrometer is secured on the stage and is brought into focus. It is then moved about until the initial division mark coincides with the initial division mark on the eye-piece graticule. A count is taken along both scales until a point is reached where a division mark on the stage micrometer coincides with a division mark on the eye-piece graticule. Subsequent calculations are made as is given below.

Micrometer Values

100x 0.01	1 mm	1x1000	$10^3 \mu$	1000μ
10x 0.01	0.1 mm	0.1×10^3	$10^2 \mu m$	100μ
1x 0.01	0.01 mm	0.01×10^3	$10 \mu m$	10μ

1. Graticule at x 4 magnification

Units 30 = 74 x 0.01

1 Unit = 74/30 x 1/100

= 0.02467 mm

= 24.67µm

2 Units = 2 x 24.67µm

= 49.34µ

2.5 Units = 61.675µ

2. Graticule at x 10 magnification

Units 100 = 99 x 0.01

1 Unit = 99/100 x 1/100

= 0.99 x 0.01 mm

	= 0.0099 mm
	= 9.9µ
5 Units	= 5 x 99
	= 49.5µ

3. Graticule at x 40 magnification

Units 61	= 15 x 0.01
1 Unit	= 15/61 x 1/100
	= 0.15/61 x 0.01 mm
	= 0.15/61 x 10µm
	= 2.459µ
22 Units	= 22 x 2.459µ = 54µ

Appendix II

Antenatals

Computer Code	Classification	Affected
1	Normal	259
2	PIH	28
3	Diabetes Mellitus	10
4	Anaemia	3
5	Congenital Abnormalities	4
6	Heart Disease	2
7	Twins	8
8	Neonatal Sepsis	1
9	ITP	1
10	Manic Depression on Steroids	1
11	UTI	1
12	Gross Ante Partum Haemorrahge	2

Perinatal Conditions

No	Classification	Affected
1	Normal	235
2	PIH	28
3	Diabetes Mellitus	7
4	Anaemia	3
5	Congenital Abnormalities	5
6	Heart Disease	2
7	Twins	8
8	Large Placenta	4
9	ITP	1
10	Manic Depression on Steroids	1
11	UTI	1
12	APH	7
13	PIH + Diabetes Mellitus	3
14	Retained Placenta	5
15		

Placental Pathology

Computer Code	Classification	Affected
1	Normal Premature Newborns	7
2	PIH with IUGR	9
3	Placental Dysmaturity	10
4	IUGR with Antenatal Conditions	5
5	IUGR with Low Maternal BMI	6
6	IUGR Undetermined	4
7	Twins	6
9	Large for Dates Newborns	3
10	Meconeum Staining	19
11	UTI	1
12	Low BMI + Normal Placental Weight	9
13	Low BMI + Small Placenta	6
14	Mother with manic Depression on Lithium	1
15	PIH without IUGR	18
16	Hear Disease	2
17	Diabetes Mellitus	10
18	Anaemia	3
20	Neonatal sepsis	1
21	Fibrosis of Placenta	15
22	Infarction of Placenta	44
23	Abnormal Insertion of Placenta	15
24	Fibrin (like) deposition in Placenta	6
25	Small Placenta	5
26	Large Placenta	4
27	Large Placenta + Anaemia	1
28	Abnormal Shape of Placenta	9
30	APH	7
31	Retained Placenta	5
32	Oedematous Placenta	1
33	Congenital Abnormalities	5

Pathology Analysis

Computer Code	Classification	Affected
1	Infarction	34
2	Infarction + PIH	10
3	Fibrosis	15
4	Fibrin	6
5	Abnormal Insertion	15
6	Abnormal Shape	9
7	Small Placenta	10
8	Small Placenta + PIH	2
9	Fibrosis + PIH	4
10	Large Placenta	4
11	Large Placenta + Anaemia	1
12	Large Placenta + Diabetes Mellitus	5
13	Retained Placenta	5
14	Twins	6
15	Twins + PIH	2
16	APH	7
17	Sepsis	1
18	Meconeum	20
19	Oedematous Placenta	1
20	Normal	159

IUGR

Computer Code	Classification	Affected
0	Morphology Only	82
1	Prematurity	13
2	IUGR + PIH	9
3	IUGR +Dysmature Placenta	10
4	IUGR + Antenatal Conditions	5
5	IUGR + Low BMI	6
6	IUGR + Unknown	4
7	Twins	3
8	Congential Abnormalities	6
9	Large for Dates	4
10	Meconeum Staining	21
11	Normal Placenta	120
12	Low BMI + Normal Placental Weight	9
13	Low BMI + Low Placental Weight	7
14	Antenatal Conditions only	18

Asokaplus

Asokaplus

Asokaplus

Authors Note

This is only an abstract and the full version is available on print and digital versions.

This is an objective study of placental histopathological findings in relation to clinical entities with special reference to maternal nutrition and growth restricted newborn infants.

Author does not claim it to be comprehensive but is an accompaniment to clinical setting.

Dr.S.B.Asoka Dissanayake; M.B.B.S. (Ceylon)

No. 217 A, Castle Bar Hill,

Panideniya,

Peradeniya,

Kandy

Sri-Lanka.

31st October, 2013

Email asokaddd@yahoo.com

Asokaplus

Asokaplus

www.ingramcontent.com/pod-product-compliance
Lightning Source LLC
Chambersburg PA
CBHW050721180526
45159CB00003B/1089